Apple Cider V

Nature's Remedy for Weight Loss, A lth

Benefits, Uses, Recipes and Lots More!

By Shae Harper

Also by Shae Harper are the following books in her "Health Book Series", these books are a must have if you want to kick-start your health!

The Coconut Oil Handbook: Nature's Remedy for Weight Loss, Allergies, Healthy Skin and Overall Health

7 Day Detox Diet Plan: Lose Weight and Feel Great – A Complete Detox Diet Plan for Living Your Best Life!

Clean Food Recipes to Detox and Lose Weight: Over 50 Recipes to Help You Lose Weight, Feel Great and Live Your Best Life!

Energizing Smoothie and Juice Recipes: Over 60 Gluten and Dairy Free Smoothie and Juice Recipes to Help You Lose Weight, Feel Great and Live Your Best Life!

Follow Shae Harper on Facebook:

https://www.facebook.com/DetoxTipsandCleanRecipes

TABLE OF CONTENTS

Introduction

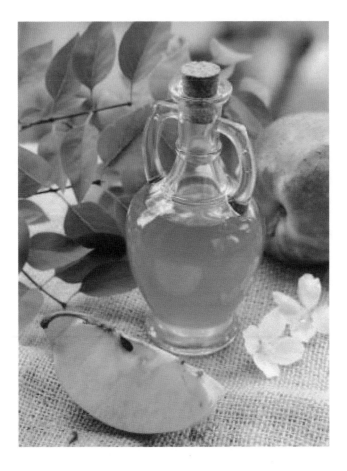

Along with cheese, yogurt, wine, and beer, vinegar is one of many favorite foods which are created by bacteria and yeasts. Most vinegar begins as fruit juice which is exposed first to yeasts, then bacteria, which work on fruit sugars in different ways. Initially these sugars are fermented by yeast to create alcohol. Then specific bacteria break down the alcohol to form acetic acid, the main component in vinegar. Both the yeasts and bacteria that make vinegar are plentiful in nature, so after the juices are extracted from the fruits, these liquids naturally progress through stages of fermentation, then acetification. Vinegar is the result. The natural tendency of fruit juice to ferment explains why alcoholic beverages and vinegar have been staples in the diets of almost every culture around the world since before recorded history. In fact, the word vinegar comes from the French term "vinaigre," or sour wine. Vinegar can be made from any fruit, many grains (such as rice wine vinegar popular in Asian cuisine), and even wood chips. In the case of grains and wood, the starches in these substances are first converted to sugars so the fermentation process can begin.

If you've ever seen homemade vinegar, or perhaps had a bottle of wine that has "vinegared," you may have seen a thick, filmy substance floating in it, often near the top. This fibrous substance is called "mother of vinegar." It consists of cellulose that results from the interaction of the bacteria with the alcohol. Sometimes the mother of vinegar is thought to be responsible for the creation of vinegar, much the same way as yogurt starter makes more yogurt, but it is more a result of the process than the initiator. A family of bacteria called acetobacters are actually responsible for the conversion of alcohol into vinegar.

Acetobacters are plentiful in our natural environment and require oxygen in order to survive and grow. If alcoholic beverages like apple cider are exposed to the open air for a period of time, the interaction of the acetobacters and oxygen in the air facilitates the conversion of the alcohol into vinegar. Because the mother of vinegar is likely to have a concentration of acetobacters clinging to it, it can be used to introduce these organisms into cider. The nature of these bacteria is somewhat mysterious, and even modern scientists disagree as to how many kinds of acetobacters actually exist. This makes the isolation of a pure strain of bacteria for vinegar-making as much an art as a science.

As cider is transformed into vinegar, the alcoholic content drops and the acidity rises. The simplest way to tell whether the process is complete is by tasting it; no odor or flavor of alcohol should be present. The strength of the vinegar is determined by the amount of alcohol in the cider. Since much of the vinegar for household use is around 4 to 6 percent acidity, the alcohol content of the cider needs to be about that percentage as well.

How to Make Apple Cider Vinegar

If you'd like to make your own vinegar from cider, fill a sterilized wide-mouthed jar about two-thirds with hard apple cider. Add to the cider either a little unpasteurized, unfiltered organic apple cider vinegar or some mother of vinegar (available at some health food stores or where brewing ingredients are sold). Cover the top with cheesecloth, so the vinegar bacteria will have access to oxygen without being contaminated by insects. Set the jar for about 4 weeks in any dark place that stays around room temperature. The best indicator of when the vinegar is ready is by taste, the only method that was employed for centuries. When the vinegar is ready, there should be no more flavor of alcohol. If you have a wine-testing kit, you can test the vinegar until it is about 5 or 6 percent acidity.

This simple household method was most likely the first way vinegar was produced. As the use of vinegar became more popular and there was more demand for commercial production, manufacturers developed a process using wooden barrels laid on their sides and filled halfway with wine. This technique is often known as the field process or Orleans method (for the French town where this method was most notably employed). With the barrels on their sides, rather than upright, more surface area of the wine was exposed to the air. To facilitate this exposure, holes were usually drilled at either end of the barrels and covered with fine mesh screen to keep out contaminants. To shorten the time needed for fermentation, other methods were developed where wine or cider was passed through a tank filled with wood chips, charcoal, or even corn cobs to increase the surface area that came in contact with the air.

During fermentation (especially during commercial production where great quantities of quality vinegar are made), it is important not to disturb the vinegar in progress. If the mother of vinegar which normally floats on the surface is moved, it may sink to the bottom of the container and decompose, adversely affecting the flavor and quality of the vinegar. The famous French scientist Pasteur, who wrote numerous articles on the bacteriological processes involved in making vinegar, was instrumental in inventing a type of wooden "raft" that would float at the top of vinegar barrels and help keep the mother on top of the vinegar. Time is also an important factor in making truly flavorful vinegar, much the same way as aging makes great cheese or wine.

How to Make Apple Cider Vinegar Using Whole Apples

This method uses whole, organic apples and takes about 7 months to ferment into apple cider vinegar.

You will need:

10 whole organic apples
a glass bowl, and later a larger glass bowl
a piece of cheesecloth to cover the bowls

Wash the apples and cut them into quarters. It is optional to core and peel them.

Let the apples air and turn brown. Then put them into the smaller bowl and cover them with water.

Cover the bowl with the cheesecloth and leave in a warm, dark place for 6 months. A hot water cupboard is ideal.

After 6 months is up, you'll notice a grayish scum on the surface of the liquid. This is normal. Strain the liquid through a coffee filter into the larger bowl, and leave for another 4-6 weeks, covered with cheesecloth.

And there you have it, your own homemade organic apple cider vinegar

Apple Cider Vinegar Nutrition

Although most commercial vinegar these days is filtered to remove the mother and any sediments, it is often these elements that give vinegar its character and healthful qualities. Sadly, many people feel a clear vinegar is a superior product because it's more aesthetically appealing, so producers comply by filtering and pasteurizing the vinegar they make. This process stops the activity of the acetobacter bacteria. The result is vinegar whose quality can be regulated and assured, but is lacking some of the vital qualities that makes it so effective for good health. Removing the sediments and mother of vinegar also reduces the complexity of flavors in the vinegar. Like refined flour and pasteurized juices that have had nutrients removed or destroyed, vinegar that is filtered and pasteurized may be commercially acceptable, but less effective nutritionally. The quality vinegar that Dr. Jarvis and the Braggs were so enthusiastic about contained all the health-promoting qualities of the apples from which it was made.

Apples are nutritional powerhouses and truly deserving of the legendary phrase: "An apple a day keeps the doctor away." They contain a wide range of nutrients, such as pectin (soluble fiber), beta-carotene (an antioxidant), and a number of minerals. The most plentiful mineral is potassium; one apple contains almost 10% of the potassium you need daily.

Just take a look at the list of nutrients below to see the potential in apples and apple cider vinegar.

1 MEDIUM APPLE (138 g)

81 calories

115.8 g water

.3 g protein

21.1 g carbohydrates

.5 g fat

2.8 g dietary fiber

74 IUA

8mg C

.02 mg B2

.07mg B6

4 meg folic acid

.02 mg B1,

.1 mg niacin

.08 mg pantothenic

1 mg sodium

10 mg calcium

6 mg magnesium .05 mg zinc

.062 mg manganese 159 mg potassium

10 mg phosphorus

.25 mg iron .057 mg copper

CIDER VINEGAR (1 Tablespoon or 15 g)

2 calories

14.1 g water

15 mg potassium

1 mg calcium

1 mg phosphorus

.1 mg iron

There is an advantage to drinking some apple cider vinegar each day that you wouldn't get just by eating raw apples. The fermentation process that creates hard apple cider, then sours the cider to make vinegar, adds important enzymes and acids to the original apples. Many people feel that these elements are important to the process of healing and weight loss. In the chapters that follow, we'll explore the role that all the nutrients in apple cider vinegar play in increasing your health and vitality.

How to Lose Weight with Apple Cider Vinegar

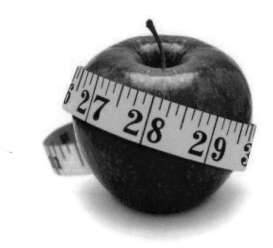

Can apple cider vinegar really help you lose weight? I believe it can. In order to convince you, let me explain a little bit about fat, the role it plays in our bodies, and how our bodies work naturally to process and eliminate it. If you understand some of these nutrition basics, it will be easy to see how apple cider vinegar can be the basis of a successful weight loss strategy.

What Does Fat Do For Our Bodies?

Fat plays a crucial role in keeping us healthy, so even if we're watching our waistlines, we have to have a certain amount of the right kind of fat in our diet. Perhaps the most important thing fat does for us is provide a storehouse of fuel we can draw on for our daily activities. We can burn protein for fuel if we need to, and carbohydrates give us instant energy, but its fat that provides the resources to keep us going over the long haul.

Besides being an energy source, fat insulates our bodies and keeps them warm. Have you ever noticed how your appetite increases as the amount of daylight decreases with the coming of winter? The temptation posed by Christmas cookies doesn't come just from your sweet tooth. There's a biological imperative driving the urge to add to your fat stores and create an extra layer of protection for the winter ahead. As an added bonus, this extra protection will provide a safety net against starvation should your food supply run short over the winter. (This is not necessarily something we have to worry about in these modern times, but our bodies have not evolved over the course of human history as quickly as our ability to ensure that we have enough to eat.) The shape and size of this protective layer is determined by heredity and our sex, much to the consternation of many women who are concerned about their shapes.

You might not be aware of the fat in your body that's way below the surface, but fats are an integral component of all our cells and provide a cushion for our hearts, lungs, livers, and other organs. Fats are involved in the reaction of certain enzymes and the activity of some hormones, as well as beta-carotene and vitamins A, D, E, and K. All of these vitamins need the presence of fat in order to be absorbed by the body.

Finally, fats are also responsible for the health of your nervous system. When they combine with the mineral phosphorus, they create a substance called lecithin. Lecithin plays an important role in creating neurotransmitters, the chemicals that work in your brain to regulate your mood, appetite, and cognitive functions (your ability to learn, remember, etc.).

Most of the fats you consume are separated from the food you eat during the digestive process and recombined in various ways so your body can use them. However, some of the fats your body needs can't be processed from other nutrients and must be obtained through your diet. These essential fatty acids—omega-6 and omega-3 —work in opposition to each other. Omega-6s increase blood pressure, blood clotting, and cell proliferation. (You could think of these as "active" responses.) Omega-3 fatty acids evoke exactly the opposite, more calming responses. It's the balance of these two functions that brings about a positive state of health. Omega-6 and omega-3 fatty acids are found in a variety of foods: flaxseed oil, olive oil, walnuts, wheat germ, and dark green leafy vegetables, as well as fish and other seafood, to name just a few.

Science has made great strides in the last 30 years in identifying the health problems caused by eating animal fats. Most of the fat in meat, fish, and dairy products is saturated fat. The more saturated fat you eat, the more likely it is that your cholesterol level will rise, thereby raising your chances for heart disease and stroke. An exception to this rule applies to the saturated fats from plant sources: coconut, avocado, and palm oil. Nutritional researchers are now questioning whether these fats should carry the same stigma as those from animal sources. Even though they are saturated, these "tropical" oils have a different chemical composition than animal fats

11

and do not clog arteries or cause heart disease. By getting more fats from vegetable sources such as olive oil, flaxseed oil and fresh nuts and seeds, you can reduce your chances for heart disease, some cancers, high cholesterol, inflammation, arthritis, and other health problems.

There are many ways in which apple cider vinegar helps us to make the best use of the fats we consume in order to improve health and promote weight loss. First let's look at the ways fat works in the body, for better and for worse.

How Does Fat Make Us Fat?

The way most of us get fat is by eating more food than we need for our daily bodily functions. Much has been said lately about the success of low-fat diets. Although it's easy for your body to convert the fats you eat to fat on your hips, the truth is you cannot eliminate fat from your diet, then binge on pasta and bread and expect to stay slim. If you eat more calories than you burn, the pounds will eventually add up.

If your weight is average for your height and body type, it's more than likely that you'll have a set number of fat cells throughout your adult years. When you gain or lose weight, these fat cells don't multiply; they either expand or shrink depending on the amount of fat they have to accommodate. You increase the number of fat cells you have when you grow as an infant and again as a teenager, and if you overeat during these stages of life, you increase your chances of making more fat cells than you would otherwise. Sometimes these cells are so full of fat already that the body is triggered to make more of them.

Carrying extra pounds increases your chances for disease and chronic health problems, such as cancer (especially of the breast, colon, stomach, gallbladder, and prostate), heart disease, diabetes, kidney disease, stroke, arthritis, varicose veins, and infertility. Clearly, being in good shape has a marked effect on your quality of life and longevity.

How Does the Body Process and Eliminate Fat?

There are several mechanisms that work to keep the body slim. Metabolism, the overall activity of the body, is one of the most important of these. It is affected by our age, sex, diet, the amount of activity we get, how well our thyroid functions, how much sleep we get, how much body fat we have, our body temperature, our weight, and our genetic make-up.

It's a well-known fact that people with muscles burn fat, and the more muscles they have, the more fat they'll burn. Unfit people tend to burn more carbohydrates than fat, because their short-term energy needs can be amply met by what they can in their daily diet. It is only during long stretches of activity that your body turns to your fat stores for energy.

Another theory of how your body uses energy and burns fat relates to the concept of a "set point." Your set point determines what level of activity will trigger the urge to eat and influences how much you want to eat. It's a natural "cruise control" mechanism that some nutrition researchers think is regulated by your fat cells. We've seen how fat cells don't like to be too thin. How comfortable these cells are with their size will determine your set point and whether your metabolism will kick in quickly or languish in the doldrums.

Your set point is also established by how sensitive your cells have become to insulin. Glucose is the simple sugar that results from the breakdown of many of the foods we eat. When the level of glucose in your blood increases, your pancreas secretes more insulin to move that glucose to the cells. If your blood sugar is at a consistently high level, your cells will be constantly exposed to insulin and may develop a condition known as insulin insensitivity, one of the main causes of diabetes in adults. As the cells become less receptive to the activity of insulin, glucose remains in the bloodstream and your body thinks it has all the energy it can use—and then some. In this condition, it won't get any signals to burn fat.

Along with a set point, there is a tendency for some people to create more body heat when they eat than other people. This process is called thermogenesis. Imagine two furnaces; one is tightly built and properly drafted, and the other has a chimney that doesn't draw well. If you burn the same type and amount of wood in both furnaces, you'll get a roaring fire and lots of heat from the first furnace. The fire in the poorly drafted furnace never seems to take off. The same thing can happen to people with different metabolisms. Lower thermogenesis can also be caused by insulin insensitivity. When the cells aren't taking up much blood sugar, the amount of heat they produce is also low.

Diets that are high in fats and refined carbohydrates drive the body's blood sugar regulating mechanisms out of balance, resulting in insulin insensitivity and diabetes. Obesity and diabetes feed on each other. When obesity is caused by high amounts of blood glucose (from overeating), diabetes can result. The condition of diabetes reduces the body's ability to burn fuel, leading to obesity.

Your body's set point can be re-established by increasing insulin sensitivity. You can do this by increasing the amount of exercise you get and eating a better diet. Whole grains and legumes, along with fresh fruit and vegetables, provide a source of carbohydrates which enter the bloodstream more gradually than refined foods. Moreover, these foods are a good source of soluble fiber, which helps slow down the release of glucose into the bloodstream. The demands of exercise will begin to reduce blood sugar levels and insulin production, eventually increasing your cells' sensitivity to insulin.

There are some people who have trouble losing weight because their sympathetic nervous system is not working correctly. This system is responsible for stimulating heartbeat, dilating the pupils, and contracting the blood vessels. If it works well, the metabolism burns fuel efficiently. If this system is impaired, it becomes more difficult to keep from gaining weight.

Another factor that regulates weight loss is the activity of the pituitary gland. This gland releases growth hormone, a large molecule which regulates reproduction and other metabolic activities, as well as growth. Growth hormone is produced as we sleep and is responsible for the energy our muscles burn while we're at rest. It accounts for much of the weight we lose at night, even though we're inactive.

There are also substances in the body that are responsible for our cravings for sweets and starches. When we eat carbohydrates, the amino acid tryptophan is released into the brain. As long as the brain is getting regular amounts of tryptophan, it determines that we're getting enough to eat. If levels of tryptophan become low, the brain will send out warning signals that starvation may be imminent. In this case, we'll crave carbohydrates which provide instant energy and a quick release of more tryptophan. An imbalance of tryptophan, especially one resulting from constant dieting, can create strong urges to eat. Maintaining a constant, satisfying level of carbohydrates will keep tryptophan levels from triggering the carbohydrate cravings that can sabotage weight loss plans.

Having good sources of fiber in your diet will help you regulate your weight as well. Besides improving insulin sensitivity, fiber can help you feel fuller and reduce the number of calories your body will absorb. Pectin is a good example of a water-soluble fiber that has a positive effect on weight loss. Anyone who has made jelly or jam at home is familiar with how pectin congeals when mixed with water. This same reaction takes place when pectin and water mix in the stomach, making you feel full. High-pectin foods, such as apples, help curb your appetite and increase your chances for effective weight loss. An interesting study on the effects of fiber on weight loss showed an average loss of 12.8 pounds over 4 weeks using 5.56 g of citrus pectin a day, along with a restricted-calorie diet.

Meals with a high fat content leave you feeling full longer, because fats are often the last nutrients to be assimilated in the process of digestion. Even though you'll certainly want to watch the amount of fat in your diet, it's important to have a source of health-promoting fats. You might consider eating more of your fats in whatever meal precedes the time of day you're most likely to feel the urge to snack. If you can't get through the afternoon without a candy bar, try adding some walnuts to your lunch. If the refrigerator is your last stop before going to bed, have a large fresh salad with flax oil or olive oil mixed with apple cider vinegar for dinner.

Although being overweight is primarily a condition of too much fat in the body, water retention can contribute to the bloating that makes your clothes tighter and leaves you feeling groggy and tired. Diets high in salt are a prime contributor to water retention, but a lack of potassium can also make a difference. Potassium acts as the polar opposite of sodium; where sodium helps hold water in our body, potassium helps cells eliminate it. If you add more high-potassium foods to your diet (such as apple cider vinegar), you'll be providing a better balance to the sodium in your foods. (This is not a license to go wild with the salt shaker. Don't make it a habit to reach for the salt before picking up your fork at meals.) *Robyn*

Potassium helps you eliminate water retention. (apple cider vinegar)

Staying Healthy with Apple Cider Vinegar

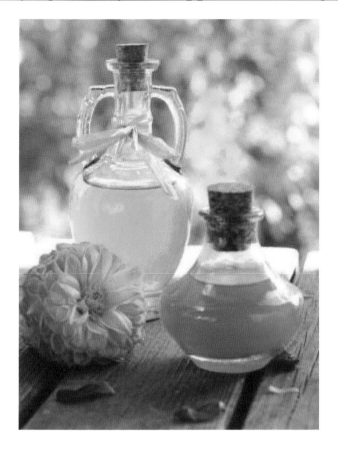

To a certain degree, good health results from a successful balance among a variety of substances in your body. Cells are constantly exchanging fluids, and the amount that is exchanged and the direction they flow are a result of how salty these fluids are. Various organs depend on the specific acidity and alkalinity of different substances in order to function properly. Apple cider vinegar is effective for health because of its role in balancing these acids and alkalines, as well as fluids and salts.

Understanding the Acid/Alkaline Balance

One of the basic properties of any substance is whether it is acid or base (alkaline). In many organic processes in both plants and animals, acids and bases are formed and work to balance each other.

There are many physicians and nutrition researchers who promote theories related to the acid/alkaline balance in our bodies. Elson Hass, along with James Balch and his wife Phyllis Balch are some of the best known supporters of this concept. Although they disagree about whether it's normal for the body to be slightly acidic or alkaline (the blood is a little alkaline, the saliva a little acid), they all agree that a balance is necessary for good health. Dr. Jarvis was particularly interested in how taking regular doses of apple cider vinegar could help the acid/alkaline balance.

The premise of the acid/alkaline theory states that foods create either an acid or alkaline ash when metabolized by the body. The pH (measurement of the degree of acidity or alkalinity) of this ash doesn't necessarily correspond to whether the food itself is highly acidic or not. (For example, lemons and other citrus fruit are acidic but create an alkaline ash.) It is thought that eating a diet high in meat, fats, wheat, and refined carbohydrates increases the body's acidity. This condition can lead to illness and many chronic conditions, such as insomnia, migraines, congestion, infections, and frequent colds. Alkaline-producing foods include most vegetables and fruits. Since most people eating a western diet tend to include fewer fruits and vegetables than meat, fats, and refined foods, they have a greater problem with overacidity than overalkalinity.

Acids are essential for digestion. Hydrochloric acid mixes with enzymes in the stomach to break down protein in the foods we eat. As we age, we don't always produce the amount of hydrochloric acid we need to digest proteins properly. In fact, getting indigestion may be as much a factor of too little acid as it is too much. Taking a little apple cider vinegar before a meal helps increase stomach acidity and can improve digestion. Moreover, the malic acid and tartaric acid in apple cider vinegar deter the growth of disease-promoting bacteria in the digestive tract, protecting against food-borne pathogens. If you are digesting your foods properly, you get all the benefits of their nutrients—and feel better and stay healthier in the long run.

Minerals such as potassium, sodium, calcium, and magnesium bind to acids and neutralize them. Since fruits and vegetables are such a good source of these minerals, they play an important role in keeping the acid/alkaline balance of the body at a health-promoting level. Apple cider vinegar can help with the body's acid/alkaline balance by providing a good source of these alkalizing minerals, especially potassium.

18

A healthy acid/alkaline balance is also important outside the digestive system. Vinegar has long been known as an effective remedy in douches for vaginitis and yeast infections. And because the pH of apple cider vinegar approximates the slightly acidic pH of the human skin, it can help restore a pH that is out of balance due to skin problems.

Strong acids have preservative power that also relates to acid/alkaline balance. Many bacteria and molds cannot survive in a highly acidic environment. Vinegar, as well as other natural acids, have been used throughout history to preserve foods, making it a natural choice for canning and pickling. Apple cider vinegar, in particular, adds a delicious, fruity flavor to pickles, relish, and other preserves.

Understanding the Fluid/Salt Balance

Another important equation in the interplay of body chemistry is between salty fluids and water. It's a basic fact of biochemistry that if you have a salty solution on one side of a membrane and water on the other, the water will be drawn in the direction of the salt solution. A common example of this effect is the drying and curing of meats with salt.

Sodium and potassium salts perform a balancing act on either side of our cell walls. Without potassium, the sodium solutions outside our cells would draw water out of the cells, and we'd eventually dry up. A complex chemical process exchanges potassium from our extracellular (outside the cell) fluids with sodium that might be in our cells. Our bodies are able to balance the water-absorbing sodium that circulates by holding onto some counteracting potassium as long as we have a good supply of potassium in our diets. Potassium and sodium also move back and forth through nerve cells to regulate the heartbeat and help muscles contract.

Sodium in the form of sodium chloride (table salt) was once a scarce commodity in our diet. We now "enjoy" a state of dietary affluence where salt is plentiful, but our body chemistry has not evolved to keep up with this affluence. The marked increase in our salt consumption from prehistoric times has resulted in a two-fold increase in our average sodium intake. Unfortunately, at the same time, our consumption of potassium has dropped. Higher levels of sodium cause more water to be drawn out of the cells, increasing the fluid level in the bloodstream and raising blood pressure.

The presence of potassium in our cells makes it more difficult for bacteria to draw moisture from the cells in order to grow and multiply. Because it works to keeps water in our cells, potassium helps keeps tissues soft. Potassium also draws excess water out of the body by moving it to the kidneys.

note (-me)

Potassium is very important for proper metabolism, as it affects the utilization of protein and carbohydrates. Unfortunately we have a more difficult time absorbing and retaining potassium as we get older. A potassium deficiency causes lack of cell growth, or, in some cases, abnormal growth. This can result in fatigue, muscle weakness, dry skin or acne, insomnia, elevated blood sugar, and heart rhythm disturbances. Severe deficiencies can lead to fragile bones, kidney problems, and changes in the central nervous system.

Apple cider vinegar is a good source of potassium, providing 15 mg per tablespoon, as well as other important minerals.

Apple Cider Vinegar - Your Personal Medicine Box

Among the experts on apple cider vinegar, there is general agreement on the usefulness of a tonic made by adding 1 to 2 teaspoons of apple cider vinegar to a glass of water and drinking this before or during each meal. You can try this simple formula to start experiencing the benefits of apple cider vinegar in your diet. Experiment with the amount of vinegar you add until you find a level that works for you. Some people also recommend adding a teaspoon of honey to this mixture; depending on your dietary needs and preferences, this is entirely up to you. And by all means, sip this tonic slowly and leisurely; it will be better tolerated and more effective if you don't gulp it down.

If you find that drinking this tonic before or during meals is upsetting to your stomach, try it a little while after a meal. If your meal schedule does not make it practical to take a tonic when you eat, try having a glass as you're getting dressed in the morning, another just before going to bed, and the third glass at some other time during the day.

On the following pages are remedies for specific conditions.

Apple Cider Vinegar for Common Ailments

Besides providing a general health benefit, there are many tried and true folk remedies using apple cider vinegar for specific conditions that you might find useful. Here is a compilation.

Apple Cider Vinegar Tonic:

1 to 2 teaspoons apple cider vinegar + 1 glass of water can add honey
Drink before or during meals 3 times a day.

ACNE - Grate 1 pound of horseradish and combine with 2 cups of apple cider vinegar. Let sit for 2 weeks, then strain. Apply the liquid to acne spots daily with a cotton ball.

AGING - This can be a sign that your metabolism is not operating efficiently. Take 2 teaspoons of apple cider vinegar with 2 teaspoons of honey in a glass of water daily.

ALLERGIES - Regular use of apple cider vinegar can help with allergies by generally strengthening the immune system and improving metabolism.

ARTHRITIS - Although there is no definitive research on whether apple cider vinegar will cure arthritis, there are many people who will attest to its effectiveness. There are a variety of formulas for using apple cider vinegar for arthritis, ranging from 2 to as many as 10 teaspoons taken with water at meals until the pain subsides. In addition to using apple cider vinegar, it is also advised to maintain a healthy weight, don't smoke, and be sure to include a variety of vegetables in the diet. Arthritis can be aggravated by food allergies, so you may want to consider removing foods that contain wheat, dairy, corn, and citrus from your diet, one group at a time, and see if eliminating any one of them makes a difference.

ASTHMA - If you have mild asthma, try drinking a general tonic along with applying a vinegar-soaked compress to the insides of your wrists. For asthma that occasionally keeps you up at night, sip a glass of water containing 1 tablespoon of apple cider vinegar over the course of half an hour. If wheezing persists half an hour after that, try another dose (although usually breathing difficulties will have subsided by then).

ATHLETES FOOT - Try soaking the feet twice a day in a mixture of half apple cider vinegar-half water, or apply pure apple cider vinegar directly to affected areas of the foot several times during the day and before bedtime.

BLADDER AND KIDNEY PROBLEMS/INFECTIONS - 2 tablespoons fresh or dried corn silk to 1 quart distilled water or marshmallow herbal tea. (The marshmallow here is an herb, not the sugary gelatin confection.) Take 1 cup, 2 to 3 times daily, with 1/2 teaspoon apple cider vinegar and a teaspoon of buckwheat honey added.

BLEEDING - Vinegar has been used by physicians up until the last century to treat wounds and stop bleeding. Dr. Jarvis believed the adrenaline-like effect of apple cider vinegar helped it to coagulate blood.

A cotton ball soaked with apple cider vinegar makes a good remedy for nosebleeds. Placing this in the bleeding nostril will help staunch the nosebleed more quickly than using a plain cotton ball. Have the person lay their head back in order to use the force of gravity in reversing the blood flow. Apple cider vinegar taken as a general tonic is good for someone right before and after surgery (with the exception of intestinal surgery).

BLOOD PRESSURE - Take this general tonic to gain the benefits of potassium in apple cider vinegar. Potassium helps balance sodium in the body and lowers blood pressure.

BONE HEALTH - Apple cider vinegar contains minerals such as magnesium, manganese, and silicon, all of which contribute to good health. It also contains the trace mineral boron which supports the metabolism of calcium and magnesium for making strong bones. In addition, boron helps elevate levels of estrogen and testosterone, which helps keep bones strong. Taking this general apple cider vinegar tonic will provide a good source of these minerals.

BREATHING PROBLEMS - (see asthma)

BRUISES- Dissolve 1 teaspoon salt in 1/2 cup apple cider vinegar. Heat this mixture slightly and apply to the bruise as a compress.

BURNS - Use full-strength apple cider vinegar to reduce the pain of burns, even sunburns.

CANCER - Apple cider vinegar contains a number of substances that protect against cancer. Beta-carotene is a powerful antioxidant that helps fight the effect of free radicals in the body. Pectin, found in cider and the skins of apples, binds to free radicals and keeps food from stagnating in the colon, thus decreasing the release of potential toxins. Take the apple cider vinegar tonic regularly to get a good supply of pectin in your diet.

An interesting research finding shows that vinegar can be very effective (and perhaps even more effective than a regular Pap smear) at detecting cervical cancer. A study was published several years ago in The Lancet by researchers at Johns Hopkins University in Baltimore and the University of Zimbabwe. In the study, nurse midwives screened almost 11,000 women in Zimbabwe for cervical cancer using both acetic acid (the primary ingredient in vinegar) and the traditional Pap smear. Researchers indicated that "the vinegar test was more likely to pick up precancerous or cancerous cells than the Pap smear."

CANKER SORES - Relieve canker sores by rinsing the mouth with 1 teaspoon of apple cider vinegar in a glass of water several times a day until healed.

CANDIDA - (see yeast)

CATARACTS - Cataracts can result from damage to the lens of the eye and are a common problem of aging. Studies have shown that people with a diet high in beta-carotene and vitamins C and E (all of which are present in apple cider vinegar) are less likely to get cataracts. Take the general tonic for optimum protection. It's important to note that diets high in salt and fat increase the risk for cataracts.

CHICKEN POX - Relieve the discomfort of chicken pox by applying full-strength apple cider vinegar to affected areas, and add 1 cup to a warm bath.

CHOLESTEROL - Pectin is a soluble fiber which absorbs fats and cholesterol and removes them from the body. Taking apple cider vinegar either in the morning or throughout the day as a tonic is an effective way to be sure you have a source of pectin in your diet. Also, the amino acids in apple cider vinegar can neutralize harmful oxidized LDL cholesterol.

COLD SORES - You can relieve the discomfort of cold sores and herpes sores and decrease the amount of time needed to heal them by applying full-strength apple cider vinegar directly on the sores until they subside.

COLDS - Your body is more alkaline during a cold. A teaspoon of apple cider vinegar in half a cup of water taken several times a day at the onset of a cold can help your acid/alkaline balance and boost your body's own healing powers. For a cold accompanied by nasal congestion, try breathing in a steam vapor made by heating a mixture of half apple cider vinegar and half water. Not only will the vinegar vapors help open nasal passages, the moisture from the steam will help retard the activity of the viruses that cause colds. And then there's the time-honored folk remedy of soaking brown paper (you can cut up a paper bag) in vinegar, then sprinkling the paper with a little black pepper. Place the paper on the chest with the peppered side toward the skin, cover with a towel, and leave on for 20 minutes. Be sure to keep the cold sufferer warm.

CONSTIPATION - Constipation can be caused by poor diet, as well as the normal reduction of digestive acids we experience as we age. Constipation can be a serious problem, as it increases the length of time that toxins remain in the colon. Eating a diet rich in fiber is the most natural and effective way to combat constipation, and apple cider vinegar is a good source of water-soluble pectin. Either try the daily tonic or following the flax and vinegar recipe from Patricia Bragg: Boil 2 cups distilled water and 1/4 cup flaxseed for 10 minutes. (It will become gelatinous as it cools.) Take 2 tablespoons of this mixture and combine it with 1 teaspoon apple cider vinegar. Drink it when you get up in the morning and again one hour after dinner.

CORNS - Soak feet in a warm water bath with 1/4 to 1/2 cup apple cider vinegar added. Rub the corns with a pumice stone, apply full-strength apple cider vinegar directly to the corn, cover with a bandage, and leave on over-night. Apply vinegar and a bandage again in the morning. Repeat until the corn has dissolved.

COUGHS - One of the oldest and most familiar home remedies for a cough is a combination of honey and lemon juice. You can substitute apple cider vinegar for the lemon juice, combining twice as much honey as vinegar. Take anywhere from 1 teaspoon to 1 tablespoon of this mixture at a time, 5 to 6 times a day, especially right before bed when nighttime coughing can disrupt your sleep. This remedy is especially good for children, who can sometimes get an upset stomach from over-the-counter cough syrups.

Another folk remedy for coughing spells at night is sprinkling apple cider vinegar on your pillow case or a cloth placed on the pillow.

CRAMPS (see also leg cramps) - Muscle cramps can be caused by a deficiency of vitamin E in the diet or an imbalance of calcium and magnesium in the body. Taking apple cider vinegar regularly as a tonic will supply helpful minerals and vitamin E.

CUTS AND ABRASIONS - Apple cider vinegar has been used to heal wounds for centuries. Applying it full strength will not only reduce the chance of infection but will also increase the speed of healing.

DANDRUFF - Using apple cider vinegar full strength on your scalp will help destroy the bacteria and/or fungus that causes dandruff. Apply to the scalp, rub in, and leave on for a half hour to an hour before washing your hair.

DEPRESSION - Depression can range from an occasional mood problem to a serious metabolic disorder. Although the severity and causes vary widely with each individual, some Eastern medicine practices subscribe to the belief that depression is caused by a stagnant liver. A daily dose of apple cider vinegar works as a liver-cleansing tonic, helped by the amino acids it contains. Since mood can be influenced by the level of serotonin in the brain, apple cider vinegar can help there as well.

DIABETES - Diabetes results when the body is no longer able to properly process blood glucose. A daily tonic of apple cider vinegar can supply pectin, a water-soluble fiber good for helping to regulate glucose levels. Since many diabetes sufferers have impaired digestive functions, apple cider vinegar can also help restore good digestion and nutrient absorption.

DIAPER RASH - Apple cider vinegar is an effective cure for many forms of rashes caused by fungus and bacteria. Use half-strength as a remedy for diaper rash.

DIARRHOEA - Diarrhea can be caused by harmful bacteria in the colon. Not only will apple cider vinegar help the body get rid of harmful bacteria, but the pectin in it will also help to absorb water in the intestines and provide more bulk for the stool. Take the daily tonic, but divide it into six doses and sip it slowly. Diarrhea that persists for a couple of days or is severe can be a serious health problem, and you should contact your health care provider immediately.

DIGESTION AND BURPING - One of the most important contributions apple cider vinegar makes to our health and wellbeing is to enhance digestion. This contribution begins in the mouth with the stimulation of saliva. Acid receptors on the tongue begin a strong flow of saliva when they come in contact with vinegar, starting a digestive process that begins the breakdown of carbohydrates. Apple cider vinegar also enhances the action of hydrochloric acid and digestive enzymes in the stomach. Anyone who is making significant changes in their diet might be helped by sipping 1/3 cup water with 1 teaspoon apple cider vinegar 3 times a day. Vinegar's antibacterial properties can help digestive acids reduce the opportunity for bacterial infection in the stomach, so world travelers might be well served by taking along a small bottle of apple cider vinegar in their suitcases. Finally, vinegar can also ameliorate the effects of a large, rich dinner eaten late in the evening by promoting the breakdown of foods that might otherwise linger for hours in the digestive tract.

DIZZINESS - Dizziness can result from an alkaline condition in the body, as well as a number of conditions that affect the central nervous system by sending conflicting information from the eyes, ears, etc. Many people find relief from dizziness by taking the apple cider vinegar tonic on a regular basis.

EAR ACHES - Infections in any part of the ear require the attention of a physician. But while you're waiting for medical care or the effects of antibiotics to take hold, try holding the affected ear over a steam bath of 1 part apple cider vinegar to 2 parts water. (Be sure the ear is not so close to the source of the steam that it gets burned.) This seems like a good remedy for young children who get frequent ear infections, as it provides relief from pain, as well as healing benefits.

ECZEMA - Use apple cider vinegar diluted with equal amounts of water to relieve the itching and dryness of eczema.

EXHAUSTION - Exhaustion in and of itself is not a serious medical condition, but it can have a temporary, debilitating effect on your performance and wellbeing. Try a refreshing apple cider vinegar sponge bath, using it full strength and allowing it to remain on the skin until it dries in the air.

FATIGUE - The amino acids in apple cider vinegar can neutralize the build-up of lactic acid in the bloodstream that occurs after exercise and stress. It's also thought that the enzymes and amino acids one gets through regular use of a vinegar tonic can help beat fatigue.

FEVER - Vinegar compresses to the lower legs have been recommended by physicians for years to reduce fever. While keeping the person with the fever warm, wrap their calves with tea towels soaked in 1 part apple cider vinegar and 3 parts water. Re-soak and apply the compresses when they become dry. A similar folk remedy involves soaking cotton socks in this solution and placing them back on the feet, wrapping the feet in towels to keep them warm.

FLATULENCE - Flatulence is a result of the incomplete digestion of carbohydrates, especially those that occur in foods like beans and cabbage. If flatulence is a problem, try sipping a glass of apple cider vinegar tonic before meals.

FOOD POISONING - The antibacterial action of apple cider vinegar makes it a good remedy for fighting off the harmful bacteria that cause food poisoning. Take very small sips from 2 glasses of apple cider vinegar tonic over an 8-hour period. Drink only clear fluids like tea, club soda, or water — no fruit juices or sugary sodas. You can also use a vinegar tonic as a preventative if you're eating in foreign countries or at picnics, anywhere the food might not be properly prepared or refrigerated.

FOOT CARE - If you've had a hard day on your feet and they're swollen and sore, try a refreshing foot bath. Add several cups of apple cider vinegar to a basin of warm water, and soak for 15 to 20 minutes. Remove your feet and air dry to increase the cooling effects, (see also athlete's foot)

FUNGUS INFECTIONS (see also diaper rash) - Use a solution of half apple cider vinegar and half water several times a day on fungus infections until cleared.

GALLBLADDER, GALLSTONES - Apple cider vinegar can be used as part of a popular alternative treatment known as a gallbladder flush. There are many variations on this, but basically whole apples, apple juice, applesauce, and/or apple cider vinegar tonic are the only foods or beverages consumed for 2 to 3 days. At the end of this period, straight olive oil is drunk at bedtime. Some practitioners combine olive oil with apple juice or cider vinegar, especially for routine removal of small gallstones that are not causing discomfort. Sometimes an enema is prescribed for the morning following the ingestion of the olive oil. The common result is the flushing of very-small gallstones with the enema or next bowel movement. While painful gallstones should be treated by a physician, an annual gallbladder flush can help avoid the formation of larger stones. The efficacy of this treatment can be substantiated by the relative lack of gallbladder problems in people who are regular apple cider vinegar users.

GUMS - Apple cider vinegar tonic can be used as a mouth rinse for bleeding gums. The action of vinegar dissolves plaque that can aggravate gums and helps fight oral infections much in the same way it does with cuts and scrapes.

HEADACHES - There is general agreement among apple cider vinegar experts that headaches are a result of too much alkalinity in the body. The fastest way to get relief from a headache is to try a little apple cider vinegar aromatherapy by breathing in the steam from apple cider vinegar vapors. Use several tablespoons of cider vinegar simmered in 2 quarts of water or equal parts of water and cider vinegar. Lean over the simmering water, being careful not to breathe so closely down into the steam that it burns your mucus membranes. You can use a towel over your head to help direct the steam towards you. Adding cider vinegar to a vaporizer can also provide relief. If you're somewhere where the steam treatment is not practical, you might get relief from breathing the vapors from a small bottle of apple cider vinegar. If you have frequent stress headaches, you might consider keeping a small bottle in your purse or desk drawer.

HEAD LICE - If you find that over-the-counter lice preparations are too toxic to your skin, try rinsing your hair with full-strength apple cider vinegar. Do not wash it out, but wrap your head with a scarf and leave it in until the next time you wash your hair. Use for 2 to 3 days in order to kill adult lice. There is no better way to completely get rid of head lice than by killing the adult lice, then examining each strand of hair in good sunlight on three consecutive days so you can strip off the lice eggs that remain with your finger nails. Lice combs won't do a thorough enough job, and the eggs are too difficult to see in artificial light.

HEARTBURN - (see indigestion)

HEMORRHOIDS - The healing properties of full strength apple cider vinegar applied directly to hemorrhoids can reduce stinging and promote shrinking. Regular use of the apple cider vinegar tonic can help soften stools and reduce the need for straining during elimination. This will help prevent hemorrhoids in the first place.

HERPES - (see cold sores)

HICCUPS - There are as many remedies for hiccups as there are hiccup sufferers, so it's no surprise that cider vinegar experts have offered a couple of options. Either slowly sip a glass of warm apple cider vinegar tonic (preferably from the far side of the glass), or take 1 tablespoon of cider vinegar mixed with 1 tablespoon refined sugar. (This is one instance where refined sugar can be used as a remedy.)

HIVES AND RASHES - Try mixing equal parts of apple cider vinegar and cornstarch to make a paste you can apply to hives and rashes. This combination will help calm the itching.

HOARSENESS - (see sore throat)

IMPETIGO (staph/strep infections) - Impetigo is the result of either a streptococcus or staphylococcus infection of the skin and is especially contagious and troublesome in young children, who tend to touch everything. Apply full strength apple cider vinegar to the skin every 3 hours; you should see results in several days. If it is a severe case, or if there is danger of widespread contagion, you should consult your physician.

INDIGESTION/HEARTBURN - Indigestion and heartburn result from too little hydrochloric acid in the stomach as often as they do from too much acid in the stomach or the movement of acid into the esophagus. Regular use of apple cider vinegar tonic helps break down protein and fats in the stomach. It is especially effective if taken before a large meal, as it stimulates the flow of saliva that promotes digestion. Try using this remedy instead of antacid tablets. Regular use of antacids can provide immediate relief, but they will overtime decrease the acid content of the stomach and possibly intensify the discomfort they were meant to alleviate.

INSECT BITES AND STINGS - Use full-strength apple cider vinegar on a variety of insect bites and stings, including bee stings, fire ants, mosquitoes, wasp stings, and spider bites. (Be sure to also get appropriate treatment for spider bites and immediate medical care if you are allergic to bee or wasp stings.) You can also use it to reduce the pain of jellyfish stings, so take apple cider vinegar with you if you are vacationing in beach areas where jellyfish frequent.

INSOMNIA - If you have difficulty going to sleep at night, try a glass of apple cider vinegar tonic with a little honey added before bed time. Keep another glass ready in case you wake up during the night. The carbohydrates in both the cider vinegar and honey will activate serotonin, a brain chemical that promotes relaxation.

JELLYFISH STINGS - (see insect bites)

JOCK ITCH - As with other rashes, use a mixture of half apple cider vinegar and half water applied directly to relieve the itching.

KIDNEY STONES - (see gallbladder)

LAMENESS - A favorite remedy for soreness in the legs comes from Dr. Jarvis: 1 tablespoon apple cider vinegar combined with the yolk of 1 egg and 1 tablespoon turpentine. Apply daily to the legs as needed.

LARYNGITIS - (see sore throat)

LEG CRAMPS - Regular use of the apple cider vinegar tonic can help the absorption of calcium and magnesium which can protect against frequent, painful leg cramps, especially at night.

LIVER FUNCTION - Apple cider vinegar has long been considered a detoxifying substance, so it would make sense that it would promote the activities of one of our major toxin-eliminating organs, the liver.

To promote good liver function, bump up the amount of apple cider vinegar in your daily tonic to 1 tablespoon. This will help to break down fats and proteins from rich foods that can tax the liver.

note

LONGEVITY - A deterioration in your appearance may be more a factor of poor metabolism than aging. Taking the apple cider vinegar tonic on a regular basis can improve digestion and increase metabolism, resulting in better skin tone, less joint pain, improved memory, and a trimmer figure.

MEMORY - Apple cider vinegar helps the body metabolize iron and provides trace amounts of amino acids. Iron helps move oxygen to the cells, and amino acids are necessary for the synthesis of brain chemicals; both of these factors help improve memory. Many experts feel that people who use cider vinegar regularly in the diet have consistently good mental powers long into their later years.

MENSTRUAL PROBLEMS - A morning glass of apple cider vinegar tonic can help reduce the flow of a heavy period. If drinking the tonic daily makes your period late, stop taking it about 3 to 4 days before you expect your period to start.

MORNING SICKNESS - Just as indigestion can be a problem of too little stomach acid, rather than too much, the nausea of morning sickness can occur because the stomach has had no stimulus to make digestive acids after a night of inactivity. Sometimes the best cure for not wanting to eat anything is to eat a little of something. Sipping a little apple cider vinegar tonic can help bring about a comfortable balance of stomach acids.

Sometimes nausea can be alleviated by cooling the body. Some experts recommend a compress soaked in apple cider vinegar and applied to the stomach in order to cool the area that's most in distress.

MUSCLE SORENESS, STIFF JOINTS - Apply apple cider vinegar directly to sore muscles and stiff joints to relieve pain. It can also be used to soak compresses or added to a bath to ease joint and muscle pain. Taking the daily apple cider vinegar tonic will help supply potassium to correct the mineral imbalance that might be contributing to aching joints.

NAUSEA - (see morning sickness)

NETTLES - (see poison ivy)

NERVOUS TIC - Drinking an apple cider vinegar tonic can help provide minerals that regulate the nervous system.

note

NEURALGIA - This painful condition can often be remedied by sipping a mixture of equal parts apple cider vinegar and water to rectify the alkaline condition that causes neuralgia.

NIGHT SWEATS - For night sweats that are a result of a waning cold or flu, try an apple vinegar sponge bath before going to bed. This might be a good remedy for menopausal women whose night sweats are caused by normal hormonal rebalancing during this time of their lives. Drinking a glass of cider vinegar tonic in the morning can help regulate toxins that the body is trying to eliminate through perspiration.

NOSEBLEEDS - (see bleeding)

POISON IVY AND POISON OAK (also nettles) - As with other itching, rashes, and insect bites, apple cider vinegar works quickly to relieve discomfort. Mix equal parts of cider vinegar and water, and apply directly. Patricia Bragg recommends keeping a spray bottle of this in the refrigerator, because the cool temperature of the spray provides even more relief.

PYELITIS (inflammation of the kidneys) - Dr. Jarvis claimed he had good results treating pyelitis using the daily apple cider vinegar tonic. As with any serious medical condition, a kidney infection should receive immediate care by your physician. The cider vinegar tonic would be a good choice to supplement your doctor's treatment if your inflammation tends to be chronic.

RASHES - (see hives and rashes)

SHINGLES - Shingles is a painful condition of the nerves of the skin. Dr. Jarvis advised applying full-strength apple cider vinegar directly to the areas of discomfort 6 to 8 times during a 24-hour period (through the night as well). This may cause a little itching and burning which will pass quickly, and it will promote better healing in the long run.

SINUSITIS - Try taking a glass of the apple cider vinegar tonic each hour for 6 to 8 hours to relieve sinusitis caused by too much alkalinity in the body. *note*

SORE THROAT (also laryngitis) - Remedies for sore throat using apple cider vinegar range from the dose in the cider vinegar tonic to using equal parts vinegar and water. In either case, do not swallow this rinse. You don't want to keep ingesting the germs that are causing the infection. Use this as a gargle or rinse hourly until symptoms subside. This is a good treatment for laryngitis or a preventative if you're going to be putting a lot of stress on your throat. It can reduce swelling and the flow of mucus.

SUNBURN AND WINDBURN - (see burns)

SWIMMER'S EAR - Combine the drying effect of alcohol with the disinfecting quality of apple cider vinegar for reducing the itching and pain of swimmer's ear. Use 3 to 4 drops in the ears after swimming or showering.

THRUSH - (see fungus)

TINNITUS - Tinnitus is an annoying condition that results in constant ringing in the ears; it may have a variety of causes. A daily apple cider vinegar tonic helps improve circulation and mineral balance, both of which can have a positive effect.

TOOTH DECAY - (see also gums, bleeding) A daily rinse with a glass of apple cider vinegar tonic can help maintain good oral hygiene and fight the bacteria that lead to tooth decay and gum disease.

ULCERS - Preliminary studies have shown that a weak concentration of vinegar can help stimulate the digestive system to combat ulcers. More work in this area may show that apple cider vinegar can help prevent ulcers from forming.

URINARY PROBLEMS - (see also bladder) drinking an apple cider vinegar tonic regularly before meals can help regulate urine production and protect the kidneys from infection.

VARICOSE VEINS - A number of apple cider vinegar experts recommend soaking a compress in cider vinegar and wrapping it around the legs twice a day for a month. Keep the legs elevated for about half an hour before removing the compress. Also drink the cider vinegar tonic before or with meals.

WARTS - Combine 1 part salt with 4 parts apple cider vinegar, and apply several times a day to warts until they disappear.

YEAST INFECTIONS - Use a douche of 2 tablespoons apple cider vinegar and 1 quart warm water twice a day until the burning and itching of a yeast infection has stopped. You can also add a cup of cider vinegar to your bath to provide external relief.

A Nutritious Diet for Health

You can pair up apple cider vinegar with a variety of nutritious foods to get a super health boost. Onions can help reduce asthma, and garlic is useful for fighting infection and cancer. Together they have been shown to reduce blood sugar in people with diabetes and lower blood pressure in people with hypertension. In areas of the world where olive oil is the primary source of fat, heart disease is relatively low. Cruciferous vegetables are real nutritional powerhouses; cabbage can help heal stomach ulcers, kale can protect eyes from macular degeneration, and broccoli (particularly broccoli sprouts) may be an especially effective cancer fighter. The lycopene in tomatoes may protect men against prostate cancer, and soy protein has been shown to protect against heart disease.

How to Use Apple Cider Vinegar for a Beautiful You

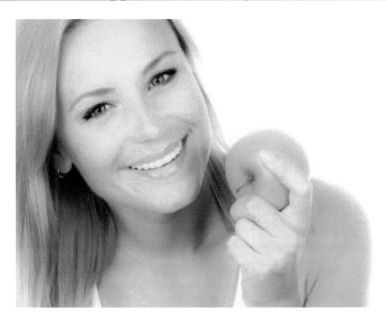

Besides being an effective tool for weight loss and an important remedy in your medicine cabinet, apple cider vinegar is also a great cosmetic aid. The surface of your skin is slightly acidic, but the use of soaps can make it more alkaline. In order to help your skin maintain its protective qualities, you can use apple cider vinegar in a number of ways that are not only healthful, but leave you looking more beautiful and radiant as well.

In the Bath

The easiest way to do this is to use apple cider vinegar when you shower or bathe. Try adding 1 to 2 cups to your next bath instead of using soap. (This is also a good remedy for sore muscles, and the combination of moist heat and vinegar is very soothing.) Keep a plastic bottle of apple cider vinegar in your shower stall, and apply it to your skin either with your cupped hands or on a wash cloth. You'll be surprised at the clean, refreshing tingle you'll feel. Apple cider vinegar is also an effective deodorant, because it provides an acid barrier that fights bacteria and other odor-causing germs. Instead of relying on perfumed soaps and deodorants that can irritate skin, neutralize the organisms that cause body odor and leave your skin with a fresh, clean scent.

Whether or not you choose to use apple cider vinegar when you bathe, be sure to try it as part of a gentle massage to invigorate tired skin and give it a healthy glow. Add about 1/4 cup to several quarts of water, and apply it to your skin with a wash cloth, gently rubbing the skin with a circular motion.

You can also make apple cider vinegar a part of a regular facial to help remove dead cells and prevent acne and other skin blemishes. Make a steam facial by covering your head with a towel and bending over a bowl of very hot water to which you've added 1/2 cup apple cider vinegar. Use a cleansing pad or wash cloth to wipe your face and remove dirt and oil. Be sure to finish with a splash of cold water to close pores.

You can also open up your pores by rinsing out a hand towel in hot water and covering your face with it for a few minutes. Remove the hand towel and cover your face with a tea towel soaked in 1 quart warm water to which several tablespoons of apple cider vinegar have been added. Place on top of that another application of a warmed hand towel for several minutes. Remove all the towels and finish by rubbing your face with a clean, wet wash cloth to stimulate your skin and remove dead cells and oils.

Hair Care

While you're bathing, don't forget to use the classic application of apple cider vinegar as a natural rinse for loosening tangles and restoring the natural luster and shine to tired, damaged hair. Add 1/4 cup of apple cider vinegar to 1 quart warm water, and use as a final rinse. This mixture will also help fight the bacteria that cause dandruff.

Another great use for Apple Cider Vinegar is for helping to kill lice and their eggs. Pour apple cider vinegar onto dry hair, coat thoroughly and leave to dry naturally, this helps to remove the "glue" that clings lice eggs onto the hair shaft. Follow this by adding some olive oil throughout the hair and remove eggs and dead lice by hand, rinse then wash off with shampoo and conditioner.

Feet and Legs

Apple cider vinegar can be used to make you more beautiful from head to toe, so don't neglect your feet. You can use it to invigorate tired feet, reduce foot odor and athlete's foot, and treat corns and calluses. For a refreshing foot soak, add 1/4 to 1/2 cup apple cider vinegar to a basin of lukewarm water, and soak your feet for about 10 minutes daily. This will help destroy the bacteria that cause foot odor and the fungus that leads to athlete's foot. For corns and callouses, use the greater amount of apple cider vinegar and increase the soaking time to about half an hour. You can then use a pumice stone (look for them anywhere foot care products are sold) to rub away any corns and callouses.

If you use nail polish frequently, try rubbing clean nails with a cotton ball saturated with apple cider vinegar before applying polish. The vinegar will remove any residual oils on the nails and help the polish stay on longer. It will also promote healthy nails and cuticles.

Finally, many of us will develop varicose veins in our legs as we get older. As an alternative to expensive treatments for removing these unsightly veins, try this folk remedy: Soak tea towels in apple cider vinegar, and use them to wrap your legs. Elevate your legs and leave the towels on for half an hour. Do this twice a day for at least six weeks to get results.

You can have the same beautiful glow as a polished apple, without the chemicals and expense of commercial cosmetics, by dipping into nature's beauty secret: apple cider vinegar.

Remember too that your real beauty comes from within, and a healthy, balanced system that is regularly cleansed and fortified with apple cider vinegar can really make you shine.

Oral Health

To cleanse your mouth of bacteria and freshen your breath, swish with ¼ cup coconut oil, melted and cooled, 1 tablespoon of organic apple cider vinegar, and 1 tablespoon of lemon juice. Do this for a minimum for 3 minutes. Do this before going to bed at night.

Cooking with Apple Cider Vinegar

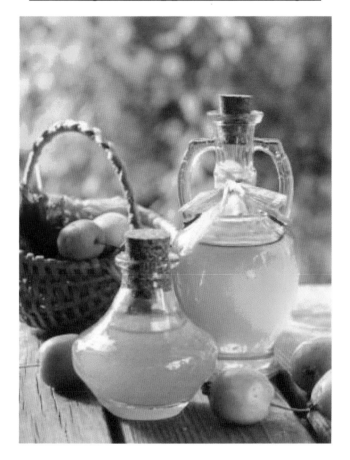

DIPS

Walnut Pate

Walnuts are a great source of Omega-3's, protein, and antioxidants. Serve this pate on a bed of organic greens, as a dip, or as a sandwich filling on Dehydrated Bread.

1 cup walnuts, soaked

1 tablespoon cilantro

1 clove garlic

1 teaspoon lemon juice

1 teaspoon organic apple cider vinegar

1 teaspoon thyme

¼ teaspoon sea salt

¼ cup organic apple, chopped

Directions:

Combine all ingredients in a food processor until smooth and creamy.

Cashew Cheese

½ cup cashews, soaked

¼ cup water

2 tablespoons lemon juice

¼ teaspoon organic apple cider vinegar

1 teaspoon nutritional yeast

¼ teaspoon sea salt

Pinch of black pepper, ground

Directions:

Add all ingredients to a high-speed blender or food processor. Blend until smooth and creamy.

SALADS

Kale Avocado Salad

Kale is one of the highest scoring antioxidant foods on the ORAC scale.

1 bunch organic kale, stems removed

½ of an avocado

1 tablespoon raw honey

1 tablespoon expeller-pressed olive oil

¼ cup organic apple cider vinegar

Pinch of sea salt

Juice from 1/2 lemon

1 carton (approximately 8 ounces) organic cherry tomatoes, halved

¼ cup sunflower seeds

Directions:

1. With hands, tear kale into bite-sized pieces and place into a large salad bowl.

2. Prepare vinaigrette by blending honey, olive oil, vinegar, salt, and lemon juice in a blender.

3. Pour vinaigrette over kale and massage well until kale is softened.

4. Top with cherry tomatoes and sunflower seeds.

Sweet-Sour Slaw

Makes 10 servings

1 medium cabbage, shredded

1 large onion, diced

1 green bell pepper, diced

1 red bell pepper, diced

1 (4-ounce) jar diced pimientos

1 cup apple cider vinegar

1/2 cup olive oil

1/4 cup raw organic honey

1/2 teaspoon turmeric

1 teaspoon celery seed

1/2 teaspoon salt

Combine the cabbage, onion, pepper, and pimientos in a large bowl. Mix the vinegar, olive oil, honey, turmeric, celery seed, and salt in a jar; cover and shake well. Pour the mixture over the vegetables, and toss lightly.

Colorful Vegetable Slaw

Makes 6 to 8 servings

I like slaws that have other vegetables besides cabbage and carrots added, both for their eye appeal as well as their nutritional value.

5 cups finely shredded green cabbage

2 cups finely shredded red cabbage

2 cups minced broccoli flowerets

1 carrot, coarsely grated

2 tablespoons minced onion

2 tablespoons sliced red bell pepper

Dressing

2/3 cup olive oil

1/3 cup apple cider vinegar

2 teaspoons Dijon mustard

1 teaspoon raw organic honey

1/2 teaspoon sea salt

Combine all the vegetables in a bowl. Mix the dressing ingredients, pour over the vegetables, and toss. This is best if left to refrigerate a few hours before serving.

Pear Salad

Makes 4 servings

This unusual salad is the perfect opener for a memorable meal.

1 large bunch watercress or arugula

3 ripe pears

1 avocado

Dressing

1/2 cup olive oil

3 tablespoons apple cider vinegar

2 raw organic honey

1/4 teaspoon sea salt

1 tablespoon tomato paste

Wash and remove the stems from the watercress or arugula. Combine the dressing ingredients and set aside. Peel the pears and avocado, and slice them thinly. (Place the slices in cold salted water to prevent discoloration if it will be a little while before you're ready to serve the salad.) Rinse the pear and avocado slices well, and arrange them over the greens on salad plates. Add the dressing and serve immediately.

German Potato Salad

Makes 8 servings

This traditional favorite comes from an old Mennonite recipe.

4 pounds potatoes (about 8 cups sliced)

3 cups chopped onion

2 tablespoons raw organic honey or maple syrup

Sea salt and pepper, to taste

1/4 cup organic bacon, diced

3/4 cup hot water

3/4 cup cider vinegar

Boil the potatoes until tender. Peel and slice them while warm. Add the onions, sweetener, salt, and pepper. Toss the bacon in the potato as well as the vinegar mixed with hot water. Pour over the potatoes and onions, and toss lightly.

Mixed Marinated Beans

Makes 10 servings

This is a great dish for pot lucks or to have around for hot summer suppers.

1 pound frozen green beans, cooked and drained

1 pound canned kidney beans, drained

1 pound canned wax beans, drained

1 onion, thinly sliced

1 green bell pepper, chopped

2/3 cup apple cider vinegar

1/4 cup raw organic honey (optional)

1/2 cup olive oil

1/2 teaspoon freshly ground black pepper

Combine the drained beans in a large bowl with the sliced onion and bell pepper. Mix the vinegar, honey, olive oil, and black pepper in a jar; cover and shake well. Pour over the beans and marinate overnight in the refrigerator.

Rice Salad

Makes 4 to 6 servings

Use the tofu or organic chicken variation to make a complete meal-in-a-bowl.

1 cup brown rice

2 cups water

6 tablespoons olive oil

3 tablespoons apple cider vinegar

Salt and pepper to taste

1 tablespoon fresh tarragon

1/4 cup minced onion

1/3 cup chopped green pepper or pimiento

1/2 cup chopped fresh parsley

1 cup cooked green peas

1 cup cooked asparagus tips

Cherry tomato halves

Green and/or black olives

Simmer the rice in the water until just tender, about 30 minutes. Immediately toss with the olive oil, vinegar, salt, pepper, tarragon, and onion, then set aside to cool. Add the green pepper, parsley, peas, and asparagus tips, and chill. Serve decorated with cherry tomato halves and sliced olives.

Variation: Add 1/2 pound cubed and cooked organic chicken or sautéed tofu.

Couscous Salad

Makes 6 cups

This quick-to-make salad is almost a meal in itself.

1 cup water

1 cup couscous

1/8 teaspoon freshly ground black pepper

3 tablespoons apple cider vinegar

1/2 teaspoon soy sauce

3 tablespoons olive oil

3 tablespoons sesame seeds

1 pound mixed frozen vegetables

1/2 cup raisins

1/4 cup chopped fresh parsley

In a medium saucepan, bring the water to a boil, and stir in the couscous. Cover, remove from the heat, and let stand for about 5 minutes until all the water has been absorbed

Combine the pepper, vinegar, and soy sauce, and set aside.

Sauté the sesame seeds in the olive oil over low heat for a minute or two until they just start to brown. Stir in the frozen vegetables and continue to sauté until heated through completely. Remove from the heat. Add the vinegar and soy sauce, and stir in.

Fluff the couscous lightly with a fork. Combine the couscous, vegetables, raisins, and chopped parsley, then toss everything to mix. If you like, you can add a little salt to taste and top with more chopped parsley. Serve warm or chilled.

SOUP

Quick Gazpacho

Makes 4 to 5 servings

Use tomato juice instead of fresh tomatoes for a low-calorie treat that's easy to assemble.

1 quart tomato juice

1 cucumber, seeded and chopped

1 green bell pepper, seeded and chopped

3 stalks celery, chopped

1 teaspoon vegetable broth powder

1/4 cup apple cider vinegar

1 tablespoon organic Worcestershire sauce

1 tablespoon chopped fresh parsley

1/2 teaspoon onion salt

1/4 teaspoon freshly ground black pepper

1/4 teaspoon garlic powder

Process all the ingredients in several batches in a food processor or blender until smooth.

Combine in a large bowl or pitcher, and refrigerate until chilled.

MAIN MEALS

Apple Cider Vinegar Chicken

Makes 4 servings

4 tablespoons extra-virgin olive oil, divided

2 whole chicken breasts, 4 halves, bone-in and skin on

Salt and pepper

3 large yellow onions, thinly sliced

2 tablespoons thyme leaves, 7-8 sprigs, leaves stripped and chopped

3 tablespoons honey

4 large cloves garlic, chopped

1 cup plus apple cider vinegar

2 cups organic chicken stock

Directions:

Preheat a Dutch oven over medium-high heat. Add a couple tablespoons of olive oil, 2 turns of the pan. Season chicken with salt and pepper, and add to the hot oil, skin side down. Brown chicken, about 5 minutes per side. Remove and reserve.

Add another 2 turns of the pan of olive oil, the onions, thyme, honey and the garlic. Season the onions with salt and pepper, and cook, stirring frequently for about 20-30 minutes or until the onions are really brown.

Add apple cider vinegar, scraping up all the brown bits on the bottom of the pan with a wooden spoon. Add the chicken stock and bring up to a bubble.

Once at a simmer, return the chicken to the pot with the liquid and onions. Place a lid on the pot, turn the heat down to medium and simmer for about 15 minutes, flipping the chicken over in the sauce about halfway through. Remove the lid, check to make sure the chicken is cooked through by cutting a small slit in the thickest part of the breast with a paring knife to have a look inside. If it is cooked through -- no pink meat -- remove to a plate and cover with foil to keep warm. Turn the heat up to high and simmer until the sauce thickens up slightly, about 4-5 minutes.

Serve with marinated vegetables or a healthy salad.

Roast Beef with Apple Cider Vinegar

2 small onions, sliced

2 ½ tablespoons of olive oil

1 large beef roast

1 cup organic apple cider vinegar

1 cup organic apple juice

2/3 cup rapadura

½ teaspoon allspice

Directions:

In an oven-proof pot with a cover, over a burner on medium-high, heat the olive oil and onions, brown the meat on all sides. Keep browning meat and turning until the onions brown as well.

In the meantime, combine the vinegar, apple juice, rapadura and allspice. Remove pot from the burner, pour mixture over the beef, cover, and put in a 325 degree oven. Cook beef for about 3 hours or until tender. Every so often, turn the beef in the liquid.

Serve with marinated vegetables or a garden salad.

Green Tomato Mincemeat

Makes 10 pints

This is a great vegetarian substitute for traditional mincemeat and makes good use of any green tomatoes you may have at the end of gardening season. It's perfect for pies, shepherd's pie and in a decorated canning jar becomes a festive homemade gift.

3 pounds green tomatoes (about 6 cups)

1 1/2 teaspoons sea salt

3 1/2 pounds apples (about 7 cups)

2 pounds rapadura

2 pounds raisins

2 1/2 tablespoons cinnamon

1 teaspoon ground cloves

1 1/2 teaspoons nutmeg

1 tablespoon grated lemon rind

3 tablespoons lemon juice

1 1/4 cups apple cider vinegar

Mince the tomatoes and grind them in a food processor. Add the salt and let this mixture stand for 1 hour. Drain the tomatoes and add enough water to cover. Bring to a boil and cook for 5 minutes; drain again and set aside. Peel, core, and chop the apples very in small pieces. Place in a large, heavy-bottomed saucepan, and add the tomatoes and remaining ingredients. Mix thoroughly. Bring to a boil, reduce the heat, and simmer gently for 1 hour. Stir frequently. Ladle into 10 hot, sterilized pint canning jars, and seal with sterilized canning lids.

To make a pie with this, preheat the oven to 425°F. Fill an 8-inch pie crust with some of the cooled mixture, and cover with a top crust. Prick the top or cut slits to allow steam to escape. Bake for 15 minutes, then reduce the heat to 375°F and continue baking for 35 minutes.

Another option is to mash some sweet potato, add to the top of the green tomato mincemeat for a healthy vegetarian shepherd's pie, and serve with a green salad.

Marinated Mushrooms

10 servings

The combination of mushrooms with apple cider vinegar makes this appetizer especially high in potassium.

1/3 cup apple cider vinegar

1/3 cup olive oil

4 tablespoons chopped fresh parsley

1 tablespoon salt

1 tablespoon brown sugar

1 teaspoon prepared mustard

1 small onion, sliced

1 pound fresh mushrooms (best if somewhat on the small side)

Combine everything except the onions and mushrooms, and bring to a boil. Add the onion slices and whole mushrooms, and refrigerate overnight.

Marinated Vegetables

10 servings

This makes a wonderful party appetizer.

Have ready:

6 to 8 cups of a mixture of your favorite vegetables, cut in bite-size pieces (You can use cauliflower, artichoke hearts, olives, bell peppers, mushrooms, carrots, zucchini, or cucumber. Cherry tomatoes and red bell peppers are nice for their color.)

Marinade

1 1/2 cups olive oil

2/3 cup apple cider vinegar

2 teaspoons salt

1 teaspoon freshly ground black pepper

2 cloves garlic

1/3 cup sugar

Place all the veggies, except the cherry tomatoes, in a large bowl. Mix the marinade ingredients, pour over the prepared vegetables, and refrigerate. (There won't be enough marinade to cover the vegetables, but that's alright.) Stir the mixture several times a day for 3 days so that all the vegetables will be sitting in the marinade for some time. Add cherry tomatoes on the last day. Before serving, remove the garlic cloves and drain the vegetables. Serve with toothpicks.

Spinach with Quinoa and Chickpeas

Spinach is rich in chlorophyll, which helps to cleanse the blood and colon.

1 tablespoon organic apple cider vinegar

3 tablespoons expeller-pressed olive oil

1 teaspoon mustard powder

1 tablespoon raw honey

1 cup organic baby spinach

½ cup red quinoa, cooked

½ cup chickpeas, cooked

½ cup artichoke hearts, cooked

6 organic cherry tomatoes

½ of an avocado, cubed

Directions:

1. To prepare vinaigrette, blend vinegar, olive oil, mustard powder, and honey with a whisk. Set aside.

2. Place baby spinach in a large serving bowl. Toss with prepared vinaigrette. Add quinoa and toss until well incorporated.

3. Top with chickpeas, artichoke hearts, cherry tomatoes, and avocado.

SALAD DRESSING AND CONDIMENTS

Homemade Salad Dressing

Makes 3/4 cup

I like the clean flavor of olive oil with apple cider vinegar. The sweetener will help you soften the "bite" of this amount of vinegar, if you wish.

1/2 cup olive oil

1/3 cup apple cider vinegar

1/4 teaspoon salt

1/2 to 1 raw organic honey or maple syrup (optional)

Combine all the ingredients in a jar, shake, and serve. Do not refrigerate.

Try adding all or one of these:

1/2 clove garlic, crushed (Remove after 24 hours.)

1 teaspoon nutritional yeast

1/2 teaspoon dry mustard

1/2 teaspoon paprika

1/4 teaspoon black pepper

Sweet and Sour Sauce

Makes about 3 cups

1/4 cup apple cider vinegar

3/4 cup vegetable broth

1 tablespoon tomato paste

1 tablespoon soy sauce

1 tablespoon molasses or maple syrup

1/4 cup brown sugar or Sucanat

1 (7-ounce) can crushed pineapple

1 tablespoon cornstarch

1/4 cup water

Mix all the ingredients in a medium saucepan. Bring to a boil until thickened.

Barbecue Sauce

Makes 3 quarts

4 cups vegetable stock

3 (14-ounce) bottles chili sauce

1 teaspoon cayenne pepper

1 teaspoon dry mustard

1 1/2 cups apple cider vinegar

1 clove garlic

4 teaspoons salt

6 tablespoons lemon juice

2 cups olive oil

1/2 cup organic flour

1/2 cup cold water

Combine all the ingredients except the flour and cold water. Cook slowly about 30 minutes. Whisk together the flour and cold water, and stir into the sauce to thicken.

Zesty Mustard

Makes about 3 cups

If you've never made your own mustard before, try this simple recipe. You can experiment with adding chopped fresh herbs and crushed garlic, if you like.

1 cup apple cider vinegar

1 cup dry mustard

2 eggs, beaten

1/2 cup sugar

Pinch of salt

Combine the vinegar and mustard in a glass bowl; cover, and let stand overnight. Pour into a medium saucepan, and stir in the remaining ingredients. Bring to a slow boil, stirring constantly. Cook until thick, then cool and refrigerate. Keeps for about 4 weeks.

Red Pepper Jam

Makes about 14 half-pints

12 large red bell peppers

1 tablespoon sea salt

3 cups rapadura

2 cups apple cider vinegar

Wash the peppers, remove the seeds, and cut into quarters. Mince finely in a food processor. Sprinkle with the salt and let stand for 4 hours. Drain the pepper mixture and add the rapadura and vinegar. Cook over moderate heat until thick, about 1 hour. Pour into hot, sterilized half-pint jars, and seal with sterilized canning lids.

Dill Pickles

Brine per Quart of cucumbers:

1 teaspoon mustard seed

1 cup apple cider vinegar

2 cups water

1 tablespoon coarse sea salt

1 teaspoon dill seed or 3 heads fresh dill per Quart

Start with cucumbers 3 to 4 inches in length. Scrub them well and pack into hot, sterilized canning jars. Add either the dill seed or heads of fresh dill. Make up enough brine for the number of quarts you're canning, and bring to a boil. Immediately ladle the brine over the cucumbers, filling the jars to within 1/2 inch of the top of the rim. Top with sterilized caps and rings, and seal tightly. Cool away from drafts.

Pickled Apples

Makes 7 pints

These make a delicious accompaniment to winter meals.

4 cups apple cider vinegar
2 cups water
6 cups rapadura
2 tablespoons whole cloves
4 cinnamon sticks, broken into bits
8 pounds small apples, cored and peeled

Combine the vinegar, water, and rapadura in a large stock pot. Wrap the cloves and cinnamon sticks in cheesecloth, or place them in a stainless steel tea strainer. (Do not use aluminum.) Boil until the rapadura has dissolved, add the whole apples, and simmer until tender, about 20 to 30 minutes. Remove the pot from the heat, and let sit for 12 to 18 hours so the flavors will meld.

Pack the apples in 7 sterilized pint jars. Remove the spices from the syrup, bring the syrup back to a boil, and ladle into the jars to 1/8 inch from the top. Cover with canning lids and process in enough boiling water to cover for 10 minutes. Remove the jars and cool on a thick towel or wire rack. Be sure the lids have scaled completely before storing.

DESERTS

Pastry Dough

Makes dough for 2 crusts

2 cups sifted organic spelt flour

1 teaspoon salt

2/3 cups organic butter

2 tablespoons apple cider vinegar

2 tablespoons organic milk

Combine the flour and salt in a mixing bowl, then cut in the butter with a pastry blender or two knives until the mixture looks about the size of small peas. Sprinkle over the vinegar, then the milk, and gather up the flour mixture gently until it just holds together. Do not handle any more than you have to. Roll out and use for pie crusts or other pastry.

Cocoa Cake

Makes 1 (9-inch) cake

1 1/2 cups white spelt flour

1 cup rapadura

1/4 cup cocoa

1 teaspoon baking soda

1/2 teaspoon salt

1 tablespoon apple cider vinegar

1 teaspoon vanilla

1/3 cup olive oil

1 cup cold water

Preheat the oven to 350°F. Combine the (flour, rapadura, cocoa, baking soda, and salt in a medium mixing bowl. Add the vinegar, vanilla, oil, and cold water, and beat until smooth. Pour into a 9-inch square baking pan, and bake for 30 to 35 minutes. Cool before frosting.

Vinegar Pie

Makes 1 (8-inch) pie

This is a basic recipe for "transparent" pie that's a Southern regional favorite.

2 egg yolks

2 cups water

1/2 cup apple cider vinegar

1 tablespoon melted butter

1/4 cup organic flour

1 1/2 cups organic sugar

1/2 teaspoon lemon extract

1 (8-inch) unbaked pie crust

Preheat the oven to 450°F. Beat the egg yolks, water, vinegar, and melted butter together. Mix the flour and sugar, and stir into the vinegar mixture. Add the lemon extract and pour into the pie shell. Bake for 10 minutes, then reduce the heat to 350°F and continue to bake for 20 to 30 minutes until a knife inserted in the edge of the pie comes out clean. Cool before serving.

Holiday Pie

Makes 1 (8-inch) pie

This variation of traditional vinegar pie is festive enough for the holidays.

2 eggs

1/2 cup butter or nondairy spread suitable for baking

1 cup organic sugar

1 teaspoon vanilla

1 teaspoon apple cider vinegar

1/2 cup chopped nuts

1/2 cup raisins

1/2 cup coconut

1 (8-inch) unbaked pie crust

Preheat the oven to 325°F. Mix the eggs, butter, and sugar together. Add the vanilla and vinegar, then fold in the nuts, raisins, and coconut. Pour into the unbaked pie crust, and bake for 45 minutes.

Old-Fashioned Molasses Candy

2 cups rapadura

1 cup molasses

1 tablespoon butter

1 tablespoon apple cider vinegar

1/8 teaspoon baking soda

1 cup chopped pecans or walnuts

Combine the rapadura, molasses, butter, and vinegar in a large, heavy-bottomed saucepan, and cook until you have a syrup that will form a hard ball when dropped in cold water (265°F on a candy thermometer). Remove the pan from the heat, add the baking soda, and stir well. Stir in the nuts and pour into a buttered pan. Make into squares as it cools.

HEALTHY DRINKS

Basic Apple Cider Vinegar Drink

Mix 1 tablespoon of organic apple cider vinegar into 1 cup of warm purified water.
Optional: Sweeten with ½ teaspoon of raw organic honey if desired.

Healthy After Dinner Cordial

If you're looking for a more nutritious end to an elegant meal than an alcoholic beverage, try making a delicious fruit and vinegar cordial. Meld the apple flavors in cider vinegar with other fruits to get a beverage with an after-dinner glow that's truly good for you.

Start with any one of a variety of fruits, such as peaches, strawberries, cherries, blueberries, or black raspberries. Sterilize a quart canning jar, and add 1 cup of 1 or more of the fruits listed above. Add 2 tablespoons of raw organic honey, and cover with 2 cups of apple cider vinegar. Top with a canning lid, and let stand in a dark place for about 2 weeks. Strain off the liquid and serve in small cordial glasses.

Special Detox Drink

The flavor of this detox drink may surprise you, but keep going. It's incredibly cleansing and good for you.

1 cup warm or room temperature filtered water

2 tablespoons organic apple cider vinegar

1 teaspoon cinnamon, ground

2 tablespoons lemon juice

Pinch of cayenne pepper

1 teaspoon stevia powder

Directions:

Mix all ingredients in a large glass. Drink immediately.

Thank you for purchasing: The Apple Cider Vinegar Handbook

Nature's Remedy for Weight Loss, Allergies, Healthy Skin and Overall Health

Benefits, Uses, Recipes and Lots More!

By Shae Harper

Also by Shae Harper are the following books in her "Health Book Series", these books are a must have if you want to kick-start your health!

The Coconut Oil Handbook: Nature's Remedy for Weight Loss, Allergies, Healthy Skin and Overall Health

7 Day Detox Diet Plan: Lose Weight and Feel Great – A Complete Detox Diet Plan for Living Your Best Life!

Clean Food Recipes to Detox and Lose Weight: Over 50 Recipes to Help You Lose Weight, Feel Great and Live Your Best Life!

Energizing Smoothie and Juice Recipes: Over 60 Gluten and Dairy Free Smoothie and Juice Recipes to Help You Lose Weight, Feel Great and Live Your Best Life!

Made in the USA
Lexington, KY
12 October 2014